Ke

Complete Beginner's Guide To Lose Weight Fast And Live Healthier With Ketogenic Cooking

ELIZABETH WELLS

TABLE OF CONTENTS

INTRODUCTION

Thank you for buying "Keto Diet: Complete Beginner's Guide To Lose Weight Fast And Live Healthier With Ketogenic Cooking", you're on the right track for a healthier lifestyle.

Did you know that being on a diet doesn't require to avoid fats?
Almost everybody associates fat with weight gain.
This is a common misconception.
Scientists have already proven that increasing the amount of fat while decreasing the intake of carbohydrates is a good way to lose weight.

This practice is called Ketogenic (or Keto) Diet. Of course going keto doesn't mean you just have to quit with pasta and eat a lot of fatty foods. To get all the diet benefits you need to be strategical, you need to follow a guide.

The fact you bought this book proves that you care about your health and that you really want to improve it. You've come to the right place. In this Keto Diet guide, you'll find literally everything you need to know to start eating keto successfully, plan your fat and carb intake and reach ketosis.
Following the low carb high fat lifestyle will dramatically improve your health and your life.

You'll love eating keto!

THE KETOGENIC DIET

What is a Ketogenic Diet?

A ketogenic diet is a diet that places and trains your body to be in a state wherein it primarily uses fat for energy. It achieves this through a natural metabolic process of your body called Ketosis that uses fat to create fuel for your body.

The ketogenic diet is done by removing most of the sugars and starches in your diet and following a high healthy fat, moderate protein, low carbohydrate diet.

With little carbohydrates in your diet, your body does not receive enough glucose to keep up with your body's caloric requirements. This eventually results to decreasing blood sugar levels in your body as it uses up glucose for its functions.

As blood sugar level decreases, it looks for the stored glycogen present in your body and breaks it down to glucose and dissolves it in your blood to be distributed throughout your body. However, glycogen stores would also eventually run out. And when it does, your body would start to use fats as a source of energy for functions in its different parts and produce ketones when it is processed by the liver.

These fats could come from the food that you eat from your meals or from the fat that your body stores. This is what is called ketosis.

Why Should You Go Keto

The primary advantage of following a ketogenic diet is that it restores the capability of your body to use both fat and glucose as fuel to meet its energy or caloric needs.
Your body is designed to use both glucose and fat as fuel.

However, due to eating a high carbohydrate diet for most of their lives, many people lack the ability to use fat for the body's energy needs. This result to bodies that have a hard time maintaining a healthy weight and a healthy body fat percentage, both of which contribute to poor health.

In fact, even if you are not overweight or obese, you may still have excess visceral fat, which is wrapped around your organs like your liver, pancreas, and kidneys.

With a ketogenic diet, your body restores its flexibility to use both glucose and fat as fuel for its energy needs. This flexibility keeps your fat cells, both visceral and subcutaneous (the fat located under your skin and on top of your muscles), in check by using the stored energy found in those fat cells.

This would, in turn, reduce the risks of having diseases involved with having high fat stores, specifically visceral fat:

- Type 2 Diabetes
- Breast Cancer
- Colorectal Cancer
- Alzheimer's Disease
- High Blood Pressure
- Stroke
- High Cholesterol
- Dementia
- Coronary Artery/Heart Disease
- Metabolic Syndrome

Other than decreasing risks of said diseases, this flexibility contributes to losing excess fat and weight in a manageable manner. Normally, while and after losing some weight, your body would feel less sated after eating the same meal you ate before the weight loss process started.

And in addition to this, you might feel an increase in appetite to compensate especially if you've been depriving yourself. However, when your body is in a state of ketosis, ketones help your body manage the hormones that decrease your satiety after meals and increase your appetite and hunger. With this, you lose weight without fighting your body to gain it back through its natural responses as to what it believes to be starvation.

Moreover, being able to utilize glucose and fat for energy prevents you from experiencing the big swings that affect your mental focus, making you hungry and irritable. When glucose runs out, ketones are readily available to fuel your brain. Even better, ketones give your brain a boost, enabling you to have better focus and concentration.

Aside from benefits for the brain's continuing function, utilizing freely available body fat for physical endurance activities that could last as long as there's fat available.

Lastly, the ketogenic diet has long been used for therapy of epilepsy. This diet has been recommended for children with uncontrolled epilepsy since the 1920's. It only disappeared from popular practice when anti-seizure medication was made available. However, unlike the anti-seizure medicine currently available, the ketogenic diet does not cause extreme side effects on patients; like drowsiness, reduced concentration, personality changes, and reduced brain function.

How To Follow The Ketogenic Diet Correctly
The Standard Ketogenic Diet (SKD) consists of 70 percent of your diet in the form of healthy fats, 25 percent in the form of protein, and 5 percent of carbohydrates.
The percentages would be based on your daily caloric requirement which is unique for every person. Since you may need to increase your caloric intake due to higher needs, you may increase the percentage of healthy fats in your diet and your body could still achieve ketosis.

Other variations of the ketogenic diet that are tweaked based on certain needs are listed down below:

• Targeted Ketogenic Diet (TKD):
This type of ketogenic diet is recommended for those who engage in physical fitness. In TKD, 30 to 60 minutes before exercise, you would eat the

entirety of your carbohydrates for the day in one meal.

The idea of this approach is to use the energy provided in this carbohydrate meal for your fitness activities before it disrupts your body's state of ketosis.

- Cyclic Ketogenic Diet (CKD)

This approach is intended for people who have a high rate of physical activities like athletes and body builders. When following CKD, you cycle between a normal ketogenic diet, which is then followed by a set number of days of high carbohydrate consumption (9 to 12 times the carbohydrates in SKD), more commonly known as "carb loading".

This approach takes advantage of the body's response to high blood sugar levels from a high carbohydrate diet, which is to store it in the body's muscles and fat cells. Having this abundance of stored energy and the body able to utilize both glucose and fat for energy, it can use this energy to keep the body going during high rates of physical activity.

- High-Protein Ketogenic Diet

This is a method used to ease into a Standard Ketogenic Diet when the weight is beyond the normal levels. In this approach, your protein consumption in a SKD is increased by 10 percent and your fat consumption is reduced by 10 percent. This helps those with obesity to help suppress their appetite and reduce their food intake.

- Restricted Ketogenic Diet

This method is only documented to be used with success for a brain tumor patient. In this approach, carbohydrate and calorie intake is restricted for your body to deplete glycogen stores and to start producing ketones. Since cancer cells can only feed on glucose, they are starved to death while your body thrives on ketones.

It starts with a water fasting regimen and proceeds to only have a Ketogenic Diet of 600 calories a day. After two months, ketosis is in full effect and no discernable brain tumor tissue was detected from the tests done.

People Who Should Avoid The Ketogenic Diet
If you are under any medication, breastfeeding, or have any degenerative disease, please see a doctor who understands the ketogenic diet. Your health could be aggravated due to your condition.

The ketogenic diet is for the purposes of improving your health and not making things worse. It's better to be safe and consult your doctor than be sorry about it just because you failed to have a consultation.

UNDERSTANDING KETOSIS

To understand how Ketosis works, you must first know how your body converts the food that you eat into energy and how it uses it. This is done by your digestive system through digestion.

Digestion is the process of breaking down food through mechanical and chemical action. Without breaking down food into their simpler forms, your body cannot use it for energy, growth, and cell repair.

The food that you eat consists of nutrients that can be primarily divided into two classifications: macronutrients and micronutrients. While micronutrients help our body to repair, grow, and protect itself, macronutrients provide the energy our body needs.

These two nutrient subdivisions could be further divided: the macronutrients into fats, proteins, and carbohydrates; and micronutrients into the vast array of vitamins and minerals.

Carbohydrates

Carbohydrates come from sugars, starches, and fiber found in the fruits, grains, and vegetables that you eat. These are broken down by the saliva in your mouth, small intestine, and pancreas into glucose, sucrose, and fructose (simple sugars). The simple sugars are for the body's immediate energy needs.

Protein

Proteins come from meat, eggs, and beans that you eat. These are all broken down by the stomach, small intestines, and pancreas into amino acids. These are used by your body to create neurotransmitters, non-essential amino acids and other protein-based compounds in your body. Excess amino acids are circulated and used to repair damaged tissues or stored as glucose.

Fats

Fats come from oils and fat in our diet. These are broken down by the liver and pancreas into fatty acids and glycerol. These are used by the body to repair cells and make different chemicals or tissues.

Vitamins

Vitamins come from the food solids and liquid that you eat. As these are broken down by your system, the small and large intestines absorb the vitamins for use in different body functions, from fighting inflammation to repairing cell damage.

These are all absorbed in the small intestines by specialized cells that pass across the intestinal lining. Your bloodstream circulates simple sugars, amino acids, glycerol, and some vitamins and salts to your liver. Your lymphatic system, a network of vessels that carry white blood cells and lymph throughout the body, circulates fatty acids and vitamins.

This whole process of digestion is controlled by your nervous system and the hormones your body produce. Your nerves cause muscles of the GI tract to contract or relax to digest food, and release substance to control the movement of food and the production of digestive juices. Your hormones, on the other hand, regulate appetite and stimulate the production of digestive juices.

There will be excess nutrients that your body won't need after this whole ordeal. Your excess blood sugar and amino acids would be stored in your body as either glycogen in liver, muscle, and fat cells. The excess amino acids get stored as glucose while the excess fats get stored as triglycerides in the fat cells. Vitamins in excess are either expelled through urine, if water soluble, or stored in the liver and fat cells, if fat soluble.

The Fasted State
Around 2 to 8 hours after your last meal, your body enters a state of fasting. In this state, your body's blood sugar drops at a lower threshold level, which also brings down the levels of insulin in it.

With the drop of glucose in your blood, a hormone from the liver, called glucagon, is released to release the stored energy in your cells. This raises your glucose levels in your bloodstream, which are primarily used by the brain and red blood cells.

After these stores are used up, the body starts to be in a state of ketosis. Triglycerides are released from fat cells and are used by your muscles and liver cells as fuel. From the liver's use of triglycerides, ketones are formed and used if more energy is needed. As your body's fasted state goes further, more triglycerides are released, broken down, and used for energy.

As you can see, thanks to ketosis, the body can freely switch energy consumption from blood sugar to the stored glycogen, glucose, and triglycerides. However, due to the high carbohydrate diets your body is used to, your body had somehow gotten used to only using blood sugar for energy.

Whenever it goes down, you start getting hungry and craving for a meal with carbohydrates. If you do eat a meal without carbohydrates, you don't feel as satisfied. This does not normally occur when ketosis occurs on a fasted state due to the ketones that prevent hunger hormones from coming out and trigger hormones that signal your brain to feel sated as if you ate a meal.

Ketosis Effect
On a diet that is high or centered around carbohydrates, your body is primarily burning glucose for fuel. Since it is frequently supplied with carbohydrates through your meals, it does not adapt itself out of a glucose burning state and into fat burning. And whenever it needs more glucose, your body would just tell you that it's time to eat.

As any excess in caloric intake would result in your body storing fat, it would just keep storing fat whenever you do. Since it is in a standard state of using glucose as a primary source for energy, your body won't readily use what is in its fat stores. This perpetuates a cycle of your body gaining fat from excess caloric intake and being unable to burn it for energy.

However, with a ketogenic diet, the body does not primarily depend on carbohydrates for your body's daily caloric requirements. This results to your body adapting to this diet and, then naturally, switching to looking for its required energy and primarily using fat for fuel.

With your body in a state of ketosis, it uses up your fat stores more readily whenever your body runs out of the fat it got from your last meal. Instead of you feeling hungry, it just uses up the stored energy in your body fat.

The Good News
There are two ways that you can do for your body to achieve a state of ketosis.

This is through fasting from food or substituting the carbohydrates in your diet with healthy fats, which is what the ketogenic diet does. Since fasting in the long-term is not a sustainable way to achieve ketosis, the ketogenic diet is the way to go for anyone who wants to take advantage of this fat burning state of your body.

However, the ketogenic diet goes beyond the ratio of

the carbohydrates, proteins, and fats that are in your meals. You must eat the right nutrients to be able to healthily achieve ketosis.

Doing so otherwise could lead to chronic inflammation, metabolic disorders, and other degenerative diseases.

WHAT TO EAT AND WHAT TO AVOID

To know what you have to eat on a ketogenic diet, you will have to understand caloric requirements and content, and fats, protein, and carbohydrates. You have to understand their different kinds and the different roles they perform for your body.

Furthermore, you need to know what macronutrients are good and harmful for your health so that you can build a diet that is both ketogenic and healthy.

In addition, for the ketogenic diet to work, you need to remove all packaged and processed foods from your diet. It should consist of high quality healthy fats, fiber-rich carbohydrates with the least net carbohydrates (total carbohydrates minus fiber) as possible.

Important:
Before you create a plan for your ketogenic diet, you need to consult first nutritionist or a medical professional to determine the amount of daily calories you require based on your age, height, weight, gender, age, and body fat percentage.

This would make sure that you are not merely guessing in setting the calories you need for your body.

Fats
In the 1980's, doctors, nutritionists, and public health officials campaigned to the public that fats are not a part of a healthy diet. They said that fat is the cause of weight gain and heart disease.

However, this is only true for the bad quality fat in food. Fats play a critical role of providing a denser caloric content per gram compared to proteins and carbohydrates. Because of this, fat can provide adequate energy when food is scarce or when a person is unable to consume large amounts of food.

Fats in your diet contain mixtures of fatty acids. These nutrients contain a mixture of saturated and unsaturated fats. Saturated fats are mostly abundant in animal derived fats while unsaturated fats are mostly abundant in plant derived ones.

Other than the dense caloric property fats, it provides fatty acids that regulate inflammation in the body. It carries fat soluble vitamins. Lastly, it provides texture and flavor to your meal, making it more satisfying to your appetite.

What To Avoid
Excess Saturated Fat
The key to having a healthy fat consumption is to minimize the consumption of food rich in saturated fats. Although your body needs both kinds of fat, saturated fats from foods derived from plants are enough to provide you with your saturated fat needs. Having high levels of saturated fat in your body leads to heart and cardiovascular disease.

Moreover, it is not enough to replace saturated fat

rich foods with fat-free food products as these are high in carbohydrates and increase risk of the same disease mentioned.

Here's a list of foods rich in saturated fat that you should avoid:
- Fat from processed meats like sausages, ham, and burgers
- Fatty meat
- Hard cheeses
- Butter
- Lard
- Ghee
- Palm Oil

Trans Fat
Trans fat, or trans-unsaturated fats, occur in nature albeit in small amounts, but they are also widely manufactured commercially from vegetable fats for use in various manufactured food products. This is created by adding hydrogen gas into vegetable oil, which causes the oil to become solid in room temperature.

The reason why food manufacturers create and use this is to make food have a longer shelf life or have a better flavor. These fats contribute to insulin resistance, and unbalance your cholesterol levels by increasing the bad and decreasing the good.

Manufactured trans fat can be found in food products like:

- Baked goods like cake, pie crusts, and crackers, and ready-made frosting

- Snacks like packaged microwave popcorn, and potato, corn, and tortilla chips.
- Fried food due to the oil used in the cooking process
- Refrigerator dough like canned biscuits, cinnamon rolls, and frozen pizza crusts
- Non-dairy coffee creamer
- Margarine
- In food labels, trans fat can also be listed as shortening, hydrogenated oil, partially hydrogenated oil, and hydrogenated vegetable oil.

What to Eat
The key to having a healthy ketogenic diet is choosing wisely the fats you include in your diet without exceeding your calorie requirement.

Protein

Most foods contain some amount of protein including vegetables and grain. Foods that have substantial amounts of protein are meat from animals, dairy products, beans, and nuts. It can provide energy for your body, however, it is not its primary purpose.

When broken down to amino acids, the body would use this to create its own proteins intended for various purposes. With the 20 amino acids that your body would need, it can create an infinite number of proteins like enzymes for chemical reactions, hormones for triggering organs, collagen for bone structure, and antibodies for the immune system.

Your body's proteins are constantly broken down and re-synthesized to build more proteins. Most of the amino acids from broken down protein are reused, but some are lost and must be replaced through your diet.

What to Avoid

What you have to watch out for in proteins in your diet is eating too much of it. The excess protein that you got from your food would be converted to sugar and then fat which would be stored for later use. It could also increase stimulation of your mTOR, which increases your chances of developing cancer.

Additionally, the excess protein requires your body to remove more nitrogen, a by-product of protein digestion, which stresses out your kidneys.

What to Eat

Moderate consumption of high quality protein is the key. Protein for a ketogenic diet should come from a variety of plant and animal sources. Meat products should be lean to avoid adding fats that are mostly saturated.

The suggested protein for a ketogenic diet varies from person to person. Generally, the recommended daily protein of 0.8g per pound of lean body mass for a sedentary lifestyle, 0.8 to 1g per pound of body mass for a lightly active lifestyle, and 1.0 – 1.2g for a highly active lifestyle.

Carbohydrates
Carbohydrates are the starches, sugars, and fibers found in the food that we eat. The sugars and starches we eat are broken down to its simplest chemical forms while, as it is indigestible, fibers just pass through the digestive system.

Sugars, also known as simple carbohydrates, are found in fruits and vegetables that can be broken down to sucrose and/or fructose. While, starches, also known as complex carbohydrates, are found in grains that can be broken down to glucose (also known as blood sugar).

Of all these carbohydrates, glucose is the most preferred as it can be readily circulated from the digestive process into various parts of the body. Meanwhile, fructose can only be used for energy by the liver and sucrose is further broken down to glucose and fructose.

The role of fiber
Although fiber cannot be digested, it plays a key role in the digestion of carbohydrates in the body. It slows down the rate of digestion and absorption of carbohydrates, thereby preventing the blood sugar from rapidly shooting up. Aside from that, fibers provide food for your beneficial gut bacteria, improving digestion and bowel movement.

Fibers also contain phytochemicals like lycopene, lutein, and indole-3-carbinol. These stimulate the immune system, fight free radicals, and protect and repair the DNA.

What to avoid
Refined Carbohydrates

Refined carbohydrates are whole plants or plant-derived products that have been processed to remove everything except the highly digestible carbohydrate in it. To refine carbohydrates, the whole sugar, plant, or grain is stripped of its fibers, vitamins, and minerals. This is done usually as other parts of the plant cannot be digested by the body or to make the plant easier to manipulate into mixtures and food products.

Refining removes everything including valuable natural vitamins and minerals and, to circumvent the lack of micronutrients, manufacturers add synthetic vitamins and minerals back into the carbohydrates.

Refined carbohydrates in an average person's diet usually come from:
- White flour from white bread, pasta, and other food products containing it,
- White rice which is usually "enriched" with the synthetic vitamins and minerals,
- Sugar from bread, pastries, sweets, and breakfast cereals
- Sugar and High Fructose Corn Syrup from sodas and other sweetened beverages,
- Fructose from
- Sugar from any other food product that has been added before consumption like ketchup and mustard.

With the fibers removed from these carbohydrates, it is digested quickly by your body. This results to a rapid absorption of broken down carbohydrates into your body. Particularly, in the case of glucose, your blood sugar rises so fast that your body would have to release insulin to signal your body to start storing it. This causes a volatile and erratic volume of blood sugar in your system. This usually manifests to sluggishness and/or hunger even though you just had a heavy carbohydrate meal. If your body experiences this often, it would pave the way for insulin resistance and, eventually, Type 2 Diabetes.

On the other hand, fructose from refined carbohydrates that are used as sweeteners and other forms of added sugars have compound said harmful effects. Excess consumption of foods containing added fructose could lead to:
- Visceral fat gain
- Increased uric acid levels leading to gout and high blood pressure,
- Insulin resistance
- Leptin resistance that disturbs body fat regulation and contributing to obesity.

High Fructose Corn Syrup
High Fructose Corn Syrup (HFCS) is a refined carbohydrate that comes from corn. It is a sugar substitute that is a hundred times sweeter than sucrose, the common sugar. Since it costs substantially less and is not affected by fluctuating import prices, it is a very good alternative for sugar. It started gaining popularity during the 1970's when it began being used by food manufacturers. Its use in different food products steadily rose since then.

The incidences of obesity are higher in countries where its use is prevalent. Add to that the fact, that in the 1980s up to the present date, obesity rates in the United States steadily rose, matching the trend of rising availability of HFCS in food products.

Moreover, studies have shown that, even in moderate consumption, HFCS is a major cause of various diseases like heart disease, obesity, cancer, dementia, and liver failure. Even though HFCS is used as substitute for sucrose, the body does not respond to it in the same way.

What to Eat

In a ketogenic diet, you must stick to protein, vegetables, fats and oils, full-fat dairy, and nuts and seeds of your diet. From these items, you will already be able to get the fiber that you need for your diet. Adding any kind of grain or sugar in your diet would only prevent you from reaching your goals in the diet. However, if you want to have your fix of carbohydrates, you can use flour substitutes like coconut flour and flaxseed meal.

For carbohydrates in a Standard Ketogenic Diet, the maximum daily intake is 5% of total daily calorie intake. Refer to the net carbs of the food items given in preparing the carbohydrates for your meals.

Beverages

The ketogenic diet is very particular in controlling what goes into your body. Drinking alcohol, sweetened beverages, and fruit juices would mess up your sugar levels and could push you further from reaching ketosis. Therefore, you must only drink water and coffee and tea with no sweeteners, creamer, and dairy. Anything else other than these three should not be drank.

RECOMMENDED FOODS

Below is a comprehensive list of the common food items that are recommended for your ketogenic diet. Each item has information of its nutritional value arranged as such: "amount of item / calories / fat / net carbohydrates / protein"

Protein
The best proteins for a ketogenic diet are those that are pasture-raised and grass-fed. This will minimize your exposure from bacteria and growth hormones. Choose darker poultry meat and fatty fish that are rich in omega 3. Balance out your protein portions in your meals with fats and oil to aid in its digestion.

- Ground beef (4oz, 80/20 / 280 / 23g / 0g / 20g)
- Ribeye steak (4oz / 330 / 25g / 0g / 27g)
- Bacon (4oz / 519 / 51g / 0g / 13g)
- Pork chop (4oz / 286 / 18g / 0g / 30g)
- Chicken thigh (4oz / 250 / 20g / 0g / 17g)
- Chicken breast (4oz / 125 / 1g / 0 / 26g)
- Salmon (4oz / 236 / 15g / 0g / 23g)
- Ground lamb (4oz / 319 / 27g / 0g / 19g)
- Liver (4oz / 135 / 5g / 0g / 19g)

- Egg (1 large / 70 / 5g / 0.5g / 6g)
- Almond butter (2tbsp / 180 / 16g / 4g/ 6)

Vegetables and Fruit

Cruciferous vegetables that are grown above ground, leady, and green are the best for a ketogenic diet. On the other hand, vegetables that grow below ground should be eaten in moderation as these have higher carbohydrate amounts.

- Cabbage (6 oz. / 43g / 0g / 6g / 2g)
- Cauliflower (6 oz. / 40 / 0g / 6g / 5g)
- Broccoli (6 oz. / 58 / 1g / 7g / 5g)
- Spinach (6 oz. / 24 / 0g / 1g / 3g)
- Romaine Lettuce (6 oz. / 29 / 1g / 2g / 2g)
- Green Bell Pepper (6 oz. / 33 / 0g / 5g / 1g)
- Baby Bella Mushrooms (6 oz. / 40 / 0g / 4g / 6g)
- Green Beans (6 oz. / 26 / 0g / 4g / 2g)
- Yellow Onion (6 oz. / 68 / 0g / 12g   / 2g)
- Blackberries (6 oz. / 73 / 1g / 8g / 2g)
- Raspberries (6 oz. / 88 / 1g / 8g / 2g)

Dairy Products

If available, give preference to raw and organic dairy products. Avoid highly processed dairy as these have a higher amount of carbohydrates than raw/organic ones. Another thing to avoid are those that have higher carbohydrate levels.

- Heavy cream (1 oz. / 100g / 12g / 0g / 0g)
- Greek yogurt (1 oz. / 28g / 1g / 1g / 3g)
- Mayonnaise (1 oz. / 180g / 20g / 0g / 0g)
- Half n' half (1 oz. / 40 / 4g / 1g / 1g)
- Cottage cheese (1 oz. / 25g / 1g / 1g / 4g)
- Cream Cheese (1 oz. / 94 / 9g / 1g / 2g)

- Mascarpone (1 oz. / 120g / 13g / 0g / 2g)
- Mozzarella (1 oz. / 70 / 5g / 1g / 5g)
- Brie (1 oz. / 95 / 8g / 0g / 6g)
- Aged Cheddar (1 oz. / 110 / 9g / 0g / 7g)
- Parmesan (1 oz. / 110 / 7g / 1g / 10g)

Nuts and Seeds

These are best when roasted to remove any anti-nutrients present. These can be added to add flavor or texture to your meals.

- Macadamia Nuts (2 oz. / 407 / 43g / 3g / 4g)
- Brazil Nuts (2 oz. / 373 / 37g / 3g / 8g)
- Pecans (2 oz. / 392 / 41g / 3g / 5g)
- Almonds (2 oz. / 328 / 28g / 5g / 12g)
- Hazelnuts (2 oz. / 356 / 36g / 3g / 9g)

Nut and Seed Flours

These can be used as substitute for regular flour in making baked and dessert recipes.
- Almond Flour (2 oz. / 324 / 28g / 6g / 12g)
- Coconut Flour (2 oz. / 120 / 4g / 6g / 4g)
- Chia Seed Meal (2 oz. / 265 / 17g / 3g / 8g)
- Flaxseed Meal (2 oz. / 224 / 18g / 1g / 8g)
- Unsweetened Coconut (2 oz. / 445 / 40g / 8g / 4g)

GETTING READY FOR THE KETOGENIC DIET

Before you even get started on this diet, you must first decide on your goal and why you're doing this. Are you looking to lose unhealthy body fat? Are you looking to therapeutically heal a degenerative disease? Are you aiming to change your lifestyle? Whatever the case may be, you must first decide why you're going to do this diet. Without clarity on your goal, you can't choose an approach for your diet and can't properly plan on how to do it.

Get Yourself Tested
You must first determine that your body can undergo the diet and the massive adjustments it would make. You also have to determine your body fat percentage, weight, and other relevant data to create your personal macronutrient mix via keto calculators available online.

Get Support
You have to talk to your family, especially if they live in the same house as you. If you're the only one who's doing this diet, your family might misunderstand when you can't eat like them or you

have a different food from theirs. Moreover, on the first few weeks, you might miss out on the next birthday party or family gathering just to distance yourself from tempting carbohydrates.

Other than that, your family can also help you in keeping you in line with the diet. They can call you out whenever you're about to slip from it. Also, if you have children, you can make it fun for them by making them your carbohydrate police at home.

If you live alone, you can get support by joining community forums online.

Plan the Meals that You will Have
Even before you shop for your ketogenic groceries, you must first know the meals you will be eating beforehand. This would save you time and would make sure that you have the right ingredients ready for making ketogenic meals. This would reduce the excuses you can think of to just nibble on carbohydrates or say that "it would just be one meal."

Also, this gives you the opportunity to research for recipes that you might like. Other than that, after you find recipes that you like, you can plan out your meals until your next run to the grocer's.

Clean Out the Carbohydrates out of Your House
This is the best way of preventing yourself from slipping up and "accidentally" eating that cookie. If there are no food items in your house to tempt you, you cannot be tempted to eat what you shouldn't. This would surely help you as the first few months are the hardest due to your body still adapting to ketosis.

Undergo an Adaptation Period

To make the ketogenic diet easier for you, you could slowly ease into it by either fasting intermittently to or cutting your carbohydrates. By fasting intermittently, you have 16 hours wherein you don't eat anything and only 8 hours wherein you can. This forces your body to enter a state of fasting and you get used to having your blood sugar into a fasted state.

On the other hand, by cutting your calories, your body is being trained to get used to having smaller portions of carbohydrates that it used to. Like in intermittent fasting, it decreases the shock of having very little carbohydrates in your diet. One practice is by limiting daily net carbohydrates to only 30 grams for 6 days in a week and having a high carbohydrate meal on the dinner of the 7th day. This is repeated for every 7 days for at least 4 weeks.

EVALUATE YOUR KETO DIET EXPERIENCE

With your meal plan and recipes ready to go and your mind ready for the diet, you begin. In the first week, things immediately start to get uncomfortable and your energy seems to have dropped to almost non-existent levels. This shouldn't come as surprise since this is normal for anyone and it is simply signs of your body being in a transition.

Common Side Effects

Keto Flu
With your body used to only breaking down carbohydrates and using it for energy, it had built up numerous enzymes dedicated for this process. Because of the body's dependence on carbohydrates, it neglected the production of enzymes for dealing with fats. Then, your body is suddenly dealing with a lack of glucose and constant supply of fats, which triggers the body to start producing enzymes for using fat as fuel. However, this would take time and not only one or two days.

This is called Keto Flu and is a natural transitional response of your body. This usually happens during the first week of your ketogenic diet. In this state, you will experience headaches, mental fogginess, dizziness, and aggravation. These ailments are due to your electrolytes being eliminated in your body because ketones have a diuretic effect. To counteract this, you should drink plenty of water and increase the sodium in your body.

Poor Physical Performance
Due to low levels of blood sugar, your physical performance will drop. This is only for the short term and your body will eventually adopt to it. However, if you require to always be on top of your performance, it will be beneficial for you if you adopt either the Cyclic or Targeted Ketogenic Diet. These two approaches will provide you the energy for your physical activities and, at the same time, enable you to have a ketogenic diet.

Other than that, you may also experience cramps, constipation, and heart palpitations. These are easily remedied by your proper hydration and by eating foods with good sources of micronutrients. There is nothing to be alarmed when you experience these effects. In fact, they tell you that your body is adjusting into a state of ketosis.

Signs that You've Reached Ketosis
- Bad breath due to acetone, a ketone being expelled through your mouth or urine.
- Dry mouth and increased thirst due to ketones being diuretics.
- Increased urination

What to Watch Out For
It is important to keep track of your ketones to make sure that your body is responding to the diet and to prevent ketoacidosis. It is when the ketones in your

body approach dangerous levels. Although it is easy to assume that ketones can reach high levels, this is simply not true and is, in fact, a rare occurrence.

However, it is still important to regularly keep track of your ketones. This can easily be done and no need for laboratory tests to be done. Ketone testing can easily be done through urine strips, breath ketone analyzers, and blood ketone meter.

WHAT'S NEXT?

In average, it would take a few months before your body can easily switch between using either glucose or ketones for fuel. When you achieve this, you can choose to make the ketogenic diet a lifestyle for you.

On the other hand, you can choose to take a break for a couple of months and get back to it just to prevent your body from going back to its old self. Either way, you can still reap the benefits of a ketogenic diet and the state of ketosis.

KETOGENIC DIET RECIPES FOR QUICK WEIGHT LOSS AND HEALTHY LIVING

Now that you've learned the theory behind the Ketogenic Diet it's time to start cooking. In this chapter you'll find 10 Ketogenic Diet recipes that are healthy and easy to follow.

All these recipes are taken from "Ketogenic Diet Cookbook: 50 Keto Diet Recipes For Quick Weight Loss And Healthy Living".

If you're interested you can buy the book on Amazon.com

Egg Muffins

Ingredients
- 1 – 2 scallions, finely chopped
- 4 – 8 thin slices of air dried chorizo or salami or cooked bacon
- 3½ oz. shredded cheese
- 1 tablespoon green/red pesto (optional)
- salt and pepper

Directions
1. Preheat the oven to 350°F (176°C).
2. Chop the scallions and the meat.
3. Whisk all the eggs together with seasoning and pesto.
4. Add cheese and stir.
5. Place the batter in muffin forms and add salami, bacon or chorizo.
6. Bake for about 15–20 minutes, depending on the size of the muffin forms.

Caesar Salad With Chicken, Bacon And Avocado

Ingredients
- 1 ripe avocado, sliced
- 1 chicken breast, (grilled / pre-cooked)
- 1 cup crumbled bacon
- creamy caesar dressing (to taste)

Directions
Tip: Some days earlier, pre-cook your bacon and grilled chicken breasts to make this salad lickety split during the week.
1. Slice the avocado in half, twist, and discard the pit.
2. Slice in half, then remove the shell.
3. Slice into about 1" slices.
4. Slice the pre-cooked / grilled chicken breast into some slices.
5. Between two bowls, combine the avocado slices, crumbled bacon and chicken breast.
6. Top with a few dollops of creamy caesar dressing and toss lightly (be careful not to smoosh the avocado).

Mexican Dip Bowls

Ingredients
For the guac
- 2 ripe avocados, peeled, pitted, and cut into chunks
- 1 tbsp freshly squeezed lime juice (or out of a bottle)
- 1/4 cup fresh cilantro, chopped
- 1/4 cup white onion, chopped
- 1 small tomato (alternatively you can use 6 cherry tomatoes, seeded and chopped)
- 1 tsp minced garlic
- 1/2 tsp sea salt

For the beef
- 2 lbs grass feed ground beef
- 1/2 cup water
- 1/4 cup taco seasoning (preferably a sugar-free low-carb one)
- 2 cups organic sour cream
- 2 cups shredded lettuce
- 2 cups shredded cheddar cheese
- cayenne pepper sauce to taste

Directions
1. In a medium bowl, mash together avocado, cilantro, onion, lime juice, tomato, garlic and salt.
2. Cover the guac and refrigerate it while you make the beef.
3. In a medium skillet, cook the ground beef over medium heat until crumbled for about 10 minutes.
4. Stir in water and taco seasoning.

5. Reduce the heat to a simmer and cook for about 10 minutes.
6. Transfer the meat to four small bowls (alternatively you can use two large bowls for two servings).
7. Top with sour cream, then guacamole, then lettuce, then cheddar cheese.
8. Finally drizzle the cayenne pepper over the top to your liking.

Zucchini Aglio e Olio

Ingredients
- 2 cups zucchini noodles (zoodles)
- 1 tbsp garlic olive oil
- 3 tbsp salted butter
- 1 tbsp minced garlic
- 1 tsp red pepper flakes
- 1 tbsp chopped red pepper
- 1 tbsp fresh chopped basil
- 1/4 cup grated parmesan cheese
- 1/4 cup shaved asiago cheese
- Salt to taste
- Fresh cracked pepper to taste.

Directions
1. Over medium heat, melt the butter and heat up garlic olive oil .
2. Once melted, add the garlic, the red pepper flakes and the chopped red pepper.
3. Saute for 1 minute (be careful: don't let the butter brown)
4. Toss in the zoodles and let cook for about 1-2 minutes, just until they become hot.
5. Turn off heat and toss with basil and some grated parmesan.
6. Pour into a bowl and top with some asiago cheese.

Garlic Cauliflower Breadsticks

Ingredients
- 2 cups cauliflower rice (cooked in the microwave for 3 minutes)
- 1 tbsp organic butter
- 3 tsp minced garlic
- 1/4 tsp red pepper flakes
- 1/2 tsp Italian seasoning
- 1/8 tsp kosher salt
- 1 cup shredded mozzarella cheese
- 1 egg
- Parmesan cheese (the powdered/grated kind)

Directions
1. Preheat your oven to 350 °F (176 °C).
2. Melt the butter in a small pan on low heat.
3. Add the garlic and the red pepper flakes to the butter and cook over low heat for 2-3 minutes (don't let the butter brown!)
4. Add the butter and garlic mixture to the bowl of the cooked cauliflower.
5. Add Italian seasoning and salt to bowl and then mix it.
6. Refrigerate for about 10 minutes.
7. Cook the egg in the meantime.
8. Add the egg and mozzarella cheese to your bowl and then mix it.
9. Cut a layer of parchment paper to fill the bottom of a 9×9 baking dish and grease up with some butter or cooking spray of choice
10. Add mozzarella and egg to the cauliflower mixture.
11. Add to your pan and smooth into a thin layer using your palms.
12. Bake for about 30 minutes.

13. Take out of the oven, top with some more mozzarella cheese and a few shakes of powdered parmesan as you prefer.
14. Cook for 8 more minutes.
15. Remove it from oven and cut into sticks.

Bulletproof Hot Chocolate

Ingredients
- 11 fluid ounces hot water
- 2 tablespoons unsalted butter
- 1 tablespoon medium-chain triglyceride (MCT) oil
- 1 tablespoon cacao powder
- 1 tablespoon cacao butter
- 1/8 teaspoon vanilla powder
- 6 drops liquid stevia, or to taste
- 1 pinch salt

Directions
1. Combine in a blender water, MCT oil, butter, cacao powder, vanilla powder, cacao butter, liquid stevia and salt
2. Blend until it's smooth

Home Fries With Peppers, Onions And Caramelized Cauliflower

Ingredients
- 1 tbsp olive oil
- 1 head cauliflower (chopped, flowers only)
- 1/2 yellow onion, sliced thin
- 1/4 red pepper, sliced thin
- 1/4 green pepper, sliced thin
- 1/4 yellow pepper, sliced thin
- 1/4 tsp poultry seasoning
- 1 big pinch of dried dill
- Salt and pepper to taste
- 2 large eggs (optional)

Directions
1. Heat olive oil in a medium skillet, over medium heat.
2. Add ½ inch of water in a bowl
3. Add the chopped cauliflower.
4. Microwave for at least 4 minutes (you can also steam)
5. While steaming the cauliflower, add onions and peppers to the skillet.
6. Cook for one minute
7. Add 2 tbsp of water.
8. When the water reduces, add one more tbsp and keep adding while the cauliflower steams (this softens and caramelizes onions and peppers).
9. When the cauliflower is done steaming, let sit in the microwave for 2 minutes.
10. Add poultry seasoning and dill to the veggies
11. Mix.
12. Add cauliflower and keep mixing.
13. Let meld together for 5-10 minutes until you

reach the desired softness.

14. Add salt and pepper to taste. (I added 1/4 tsp salt, pepper to taste)

15. Optional: If you want you can split into two servings and top with sunny-side up eggs.

Unbaked Strawberry Muffin

Ingredients
- 1 oz. cream cheese
- 1 tbsp unsalted butter
- 1 tbsp Steviva Blend + 1 tbsp hot water, mixed (or 2 tbsp sugar-free vanilla syrup)
- 1/2 tsp vanilla extract
- 1 tbsp coconut flour
- 2 tbsp almond flour
- 3 strawberries (chopped)

Directions
1. In a mug, melt the cream cheese and butter in the microwave or in a saucepan.
2. Add hot water, Steviva Blend and vanilla extract.
3. Mix it.
4. Add coconut flour and almond flour and mix it again.
5. Add in the chopped strawberries and mix into a dough.

Ketoproof Coffee

Ingredients
- 2 cups coffee
- 2 tbsp. grass fed unsalted butter
- 2 tbsp. organic coconut oil (or MCT oil)
- 1 tbsp. heavy cream (optional)
- 1 tsp. vanilla extract (optional)

Directions
1. Brew 2 cups of coffee into a large container with your favorite method. (Choose something large enough to eliminate spilling when you'll blend it).
2. Fill the coffee filter and wet the coffee with a little bit of water, allowing about 30 seconds for it to "bloom".
3. Brew normally by pouring the water in a circular motion, (make sure the coffee isn't swimming in water).
4. Grab the butter, coconut oil, and immersion blender.
5. Cut off 2 tbsp. of grass fed butter.
6. Drop in the butter, then add 1 tsp. of vanilla extract, and plunk in the 2 tbsp. of coconut oil (or MCT oil).
7. Add 1 tbsp. of heavy cream.
8. Mix it with the immersion blender for about 45-60 (move the immersion blender up and down to emulsify all of the fat into the coffee and aerate the mixture)
9. Pour it in a mug and drink it.

No Bake Chocolate Mousse Tart

Ingredients
For the crust:
- 1 1/4 cups almond flour
- 1/4 cup cocoa powder
- 1/4 cup powdered Swerve Sweetener
- 5 tbsp butter, melted

For the chocolate Mousse Filling:
- 3/4 cup whipping cream
- 3/4 cup unsweetened almond or cashew milk
- 1/4 cup butter
- 3 ounces good quality unsweetened dark chocolate, chopped (do not use sweetened chocolate here, as your mousse may not set properly)
- 3 tbsp cocoa powder
- 6 tbsp powdered Swerve Sweetener
- 1/2 tsp espresso powder (optional, boosts chocolate flavour)
- 3 large eggs

For the topping:
- 1 cup whipping cream
- 2 tbsp powdered Swerve Sweetener
- 1/4 tsp vanilla extract
- 1/2 ounce dark sugar-free chocolate

Directions
For the crust:
1. Slightly grease a 9 inch tart pan with a removable bottom.
2. In a medium bowl, whisk together the cocoa powder, almond flour and the sweetener.
3. Add the melted butter and stir it until the mixture clumps together.

4. Press firmly into bottom and up sides of the prepared tart pan.
5. Refrigerate it until the filling is ready.

For the chocolate Mousse:
1. In a small pan, combine almond or cashew milk, cream and butter.
2. Bring it to a full boil and then remove it from the heat.
3. In a blender, combine the unsweetened chocolate, the cocoa powder, the espresso powder and the sweetener.
4. Pour the scalded cream in the mixture and blend until it's smooth.
5. Add the eggs and blend again until it's smooth.
6. Pour into the chilled crust and chill until firm, for at least 1 hour.
7. Gently press the tart pan from the bottom to remove sides and place on the serving platter.

For the topping:
1. Beat some whipping cream with sweetener and vanilla until it holds stiff peaks.
2. Spread over the mousse to the edges of your tart.
3. Use a cheese grater to shave some dark chocolate over the whipping cream.
4. Let it set a bit in the refrigerator, then serve.

OTHER BOOKS BY ELIZABETH WELLS

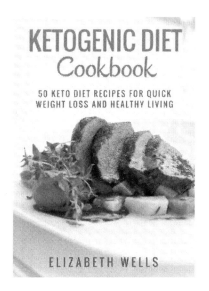

Did you enjoy these keto dishes?

"Ketogenic Diet Cookbook" contains these and other keto recipes that can definitely improve your eating habits and your life. You'll learn how to craft healthy keto breakfasts and how to cook delicious low carb dishes for lunch and dinner. You'll also find recipes to prepare tasty keto desserts.

Here are some recipes you'll learn:

- Keto Pizza Rolls
- Low Carb Mocha Chia Pudding
- Ketogenic Italian Parmesan Breaded Pork Cutlets
- Pancakes With Cinnamon
- Keto Chocolate Mousse
- Swedish Meatballs
- And much more

Cooking keto is easy, if you follow the right recipes. What are you waiting for? Start cooking healthier today!

You can find "Ketogenic Diet Cookbook: 50 Keto Diet Recipes For Quick Weight Loss And Healthy Living" on Amazon.com

CONCLUSION

I hope this guide has helped you eat healthier and lose weight by achieving ketosis.
The keto world is constantly growing, and everyday more and more people are discovering this amazing lifestyle.

Your support is always welcome, if you enjoyed these recipes, please take the time to share your thoughts and post a review on Amazon to help other people eat healthier. It'd be greatly appreciated!

Thank you again and good luck with your keto diet experience.

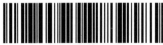

Made in the USA
San Bernardino, CA
07 June 2017